LEAN AND GREEN RECIPES FOR BEGINNERS 2021

Tasty, Lean and Green Recipes to Lose Weight Fast and Enjoy Scrumptious Food Without Feeling Hungry

Gwenda Smith

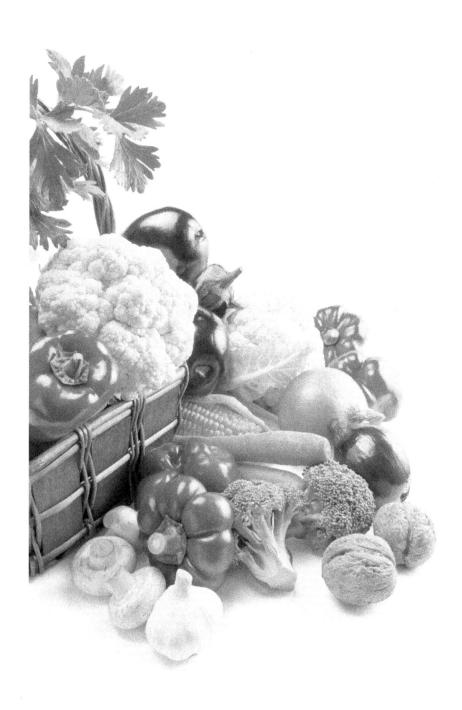

TABLE OF CONTENT

INTRODUCTION 9

LEAN AND GREEN DIET BENEFITS 10

FOOD TO EAT AND TO AVOID 11

BREAKFAST 17

    ALKALINE BLUEBERRY MUFFINS 18

    CRUNCHY QUINOA MEAL 20

    COCONUT PANCAKES 22

    QUINOA PORRIDGE 24

    BANANA BARLEY PORRIDGE 26

    ZUCCHINI MUFFINS 28

LUNCH 31

    CHICKEN LOAF 32

    CHICKEN STROGANOFF 34

    LEMON CAPER PESTO 36

    BACON SPAGHETTI SQUASH CARBONARA 37

    BUTTERED BAKED COD WITH WINE 39

    SPICED SORGHUM AND BERRIES 41

    GREEK SALAD 43

    GRILLED EGGPLANTS 45

    ASPARAGUS AVOCADO SOUP 47

    BEER BATTERED COD FILET 49

    SWEET POTATO CHIPS 51

Easy Beef Mushroom Stew	53
Béarnaise Sauce	55
Butterflied Prawns with Garlic-Sriracha	57
Chili Sauce	59
Vanilla Caramel Sauce	61
Buffalo Chicken Soup	62
Cajun Seasoned Salmon Filet	64
Chicken Fillets with Artichoke Hearts	66
Chicken Meatballs with Carrot	68
Buttered Garlic-Oregano on Clams	70

DINNER 73

Thyme Scallops	74
Oregano Pork Mix	76
Simple Beef Roast	78
Chicken Breast Soup	80
Cauliflower Curry	81
Tender & Juicy Lamb Roast	82
Basil Cheese Pork Roast	84
Feta Lamb Patties	86
Beef Stroganoff	88
Eggplant and Carrots Mix	90
Parmesan Eggplants	91
Kale Sauté	92
Carrots Sauté	93

DESSERT 96

- ALMONDS AND OATS PUDDING 97
- STRAWBERRY SORBET 98
- CHOCOLATE FONDUE 100
- RICE PUDDING 102
- BRAISED APPLES 104
- WINE FIGS 105
- OLIVES AND CHEESE STUFFED TOMATOES 107
- TOMATO SALSA 108
- CHILI MANGO AND WATERMELON SALSA 110
- APPLE KALE CUCUMBER SMOOTHIE 112
- COCOA CAKE 114
- APPLE BREAD 116

CONCLUSION 119

© **Copyright 2021 by Gwenda Smith - All rights reserved.**

The following Book is reproduced below with the goal of providing information that is as accurate and reliable as possible. Regardless, purchasing this Book can be seen as consent to the fact that both the publisher and the author of this book are in no way experts on the topics discussed within and that any recommendations or suggestions that are made herein are for entertainment purposes only. Professionals should be consulted as needed prior to undertaking any of the action endorsed herein.

This declaration is deemed fair and valid by both the American Bar Association and the Committee of Publishers Association and is legally binding throughout the United States.

Furthermore, the transmission, duplication, or reproduction of any of the following work including specific information will be considered an illegal act irrespective of if it is done electronically or in print. This extends to creating a secondary or tertiary copy of the work or a recorded copy and is only allowed with the express written consent from the Publisher. All additional right reserved.

The information in the following pages is broadly considered a truthful and accurate account of facts and as such, any inattention, use, or misuse of the information in question by the reader will render any resulting actions solely under their purview. There are no scenarios in which the publisher or the original author of this work can be in any fashion deemed liable for any hardship or damages that may befall them after undertaking information described herein.

Additionally, the information in the following pages is intended only for informational purposes and should thus be thought of as universal. As befitting its nature, it is presented without assurance regarding its prolonged validity or interim quality. Trademarks that are mentioned are done without written consent and can in no way be considered an endorsement from the trademark holder.

INTRODUCTION

The Lean and Green diet is a brand-new eating program, it is very detailed and fits the needs of people who want to prepare healthy dishes for themselves and their families, reducing modern-day consumerism and improving their quality of life and will also help you lose those excess pounds.

The Lean and Green Diet was designed for anyone who wants to lose weight and feel good about themselves through healthy eating. As you lose weight with this regimen, you can feel better about yourself with a positive self-image. After losing weight, you will have more energy and be less likely to get sick as well.

The Lean and Green Diet's unique nutrition concept has helped millions of people across the world lose weight and improve their health!

So, let 's discover more and learn delicious recipes from breakfast to dessert and let the Lean and Green diet be your partner in weight loss!

LEAN AND GREEN DIET BENEFITS

Lean and green meals may be a solid match for you on the off chance that you need a diet plan that is clear and simple to follow, that will assist you with getting in shape rapidly, and offers worked in social help. Below are the reasons why this diet regimen is considered as the easiest to follow among all commercial diet regimens.

Accomplishes Rapid Weight Loss

Most individuals require around 1600 to 3000 calories for each day to keep up their weight. Limiting that number to as low as 800 basically ensures weight loss for a great many people.

Easy to Follow

You are encouraged to prepare 1 to 3 green and lean foods a day, depending on your strategy, they are very simple to prepare, as the program will include detailed recipes and a list of food options to choose from.

No Counting Calories

You don't really need to count your calories when following this type of diet, just as long as you stick with the rule of fuelings, meals, snacks and water intake depending on your preference.

FOOD TO EAT AND TO AVOID

There are a lot many foods that you can eat however, you must know them by heart, and this is particularly true if you are just new to this diet. This section is dedicated to the types of foods that are recommended and those to avoid while following this diet regimen.

FOOD TO EAT

There are numerous categories of foods that can be eaten under this diet regimen. This section will break down the Lean and Green foods that you can eat while following this diet regime.

Lean Foods

Leanest Foods - These foods are considered to be the leanest as it has only up to 4 grams of total fat. Moreover, dieters should eat a 7-ounce cooked portion of these foods. Consume these foods with 1 healthy fat serving.

Fish: Flounder, cod, haddock, grouper, Mahi, tilapia, tuna (yellowfin fresh or canned), and wild catfish.

Shellfish: Scallops, lobster, crabs, shrimp

Game meat: Elk, deer, buffalo

Ground turkey or other meat: Should be 98% lean

Meatless alternatives: 14 egg whites, 2 cups egg substitute, 5 ounces seitan, 1 ½ cups 1% cottage cheese, and 12 ounces non-fat 0% Greek yogurt

Leaner Foods - These foods contain 5 to 9 grams of total fat. Consume these foods with 1 healthy fat serving. Make sure to consume only 6 ounces of a cooked portion of these foods daily:

Fish: Halibut, trout, and swordfish

Chicken: White meat such as breasts as long as the skin is removed

Turkey: Ground turkey as long as it is 95% to 97% lean.

Meatless options: 2 whole eggs plus 4 egg whites, 2 whole eggs plus one cup egg substitute, 1 ½ cups 2% cottage cheese, and 12 ounces low fat 2% plain Greek yogurt

Lean Foods - These are foods that contain 10g to 20g total fat. When consuming these foods, there should be no serving of healthy fat. These include the following:

Fish: Tuna (bluefin steak), salmon, herring, farmed catfish, and mackerel

Lean beef: Ground, steak, and roast

Lamb: All cuts

Pork: Pork chops, pork tenderloin, and all parts. Make sure to remove the skin

Ground turkey and other meats: 85% to 94% lean

Chicken: Any dark meat

Meatless options: 15 ounces extra-firm tofu, 3 whole eggs (up to two times per week), 4 ounces reduced-fat skim cheese, 8 ounces part-skim ricotta cheese, and 5 ounces tempeh

Healthy Fat Servings - Healthy fat servings are allowed under this diet. They should contain 5 grams of fat and less than 5 grams of carbohydrates. Make sure that you add between 0 and 2 healthy fat servings daily. Below are the different healthy fat servings that you can eat:

1 teaspoon oil (any kind of oil)

1 tablespoon low carbohydrate salad dressing

2 tablespoons reduced-fat salad dressing

5 to 10 black or green olives

1 ½ ounce avocado

1/3-ounce plain nuts including peanuts, almonds, pistachios

1 tablespoon plain seeds such as chia, sesame, flax, and pumpkin seeds

½ tablespoon regular butter, mayonnaise, and margarine

Green Foods

This section will discuss the green servings that you still need to consume.

These include all kinds of vegetables that have been categorized from lower, moderate, and high in terms of carbohydrate content. One serving of vegetables should be at ½ cup unless otherwise specified.

Lower Carbohydrate - These are vegetables that contain low amounts of carbohydrates.

A cup of green leafy vegetables, such as collard greens (raw), lettuce (green leaf, iceberg, butterhead, and romaine), spinach (raw), mustard greens, spring mix, bok choy (raw), and watercress.

½ cup of vegetables including cucumbers, celery, radishes, white mushroom, sprouts (mung bean, alfalfa), arugula, turnip greens, escarole, nopales, Swiss chard (raw), jalapeno, and bok choy (cooked).

Moderate Carbohydrate - These are vegetables that contain moderate amounts of carbohydrates. Below are the types of vegetables that can be consumed in moderation:

½ cup of any of the following vegetables such as asparagus, cauliflower, fennel bulb, eggplant, portabella mushrooms, kale, cooked spinach, summer squash (zucchini and scallop).

Higher Carbohydrates - Foods that are under this category contain a high amount of starch. Make sure to consume limited amounts of these vegetables.

½ cup of the following vegetables like chayote squash, red cabbage, broccoli, cooked collard and mustard greens, green or wax beans, kohlrabi, kabocha squash, cooked leeks, any peppers, okra, raw scallion, summer squash such as straight neck and crookneck, tomatoes, spaghetti squash, turnips, jicama, cooked Swiss chard, and hearts of palm.

FOODS TO AVOID

The following foods are to be avoided; except it's included in the fueling they include:

- Fried foods: meats, fish, shellfish, vegetables, desserts like baked goods
- Refined grains: white bread, pasta, scones, hotcakes, flour tortillas, wafers, white rice, treats, cakes, cakes
- Certain fats: margarine, coconut oil, strong shortening
- Whole fat dairy: milk, cheddar, yogurt
- Alcohol: all varieties, no exception
- Sugar-sweetened beverages: pop, natural product juice, sports drinks, caffeinated drinks, sweet tea

BREAKFAST

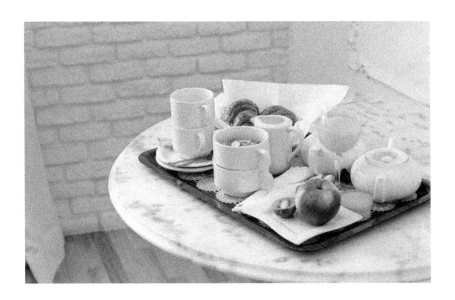

Alkaline Blueberry Muffins

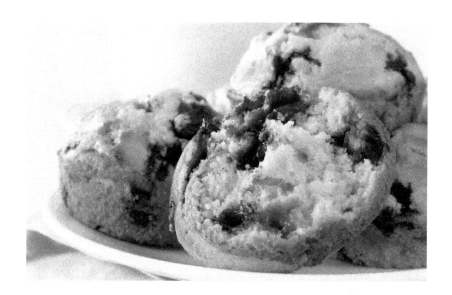

Preparation Time: 5 Minutes

Cooking Time: 20 minutes

Servings: 3

Ingredients:

- 1 cup Coconut Milk
- 3/4 cup Spelt Flour
- 3/4 Teff Flour
- 1/2 cup Blueberries
- 1/3 cup Agave
- 1/4 cup Sea Moss Gel
- 1/2 tsp. Sea Salt
- Grapeseed Oil

Directions:

1. Adjust the temperature of the oven to 365 °F.
2. Grease 6 regular-size muffin cups with muffin liners.
3. In a bowl, mix together sea salt, sea moss, agave, coconut milk, and flour gel until they are properly blended.
4. You then crimp in blueberries.
5. Coat the muffin pan lightly with the grapeseed oil.
6. Pour in the muffin batter.
7. Bake for at least 30 minutes until it turns golden brown.
8. Serve.

Nutrition:

Calories: 160 kcal

Fat: 5g

Carbs: 25g

Proteins: 2g

Crunchy Quinoa Meal

Preparation Time: 5 minutes

Cooking Time: 25 minutes

Servings: 2

Ingredients:

- 3 cups coconut milk
- 1 cup rinsed quinoa
- 1/8 tsp. ground cinnamon
- 1 cup raspberry
- 1/2 cup chopped coconuts

Directions:

1. In a saucepan, pour milk and bring to a boil over moderate heat.
2. Add the quinoa to the milk and then bring it to a boil once more.
3. You then let it simmer for at least 15 minutes on medium heat until the milk is reduced.
4. Stir in the cinnamon then mix properly.
5. Cover it then cook for 8 minutes until the milk is completely absorbed.
6. Add the raspberry and cook the meal for 30 seconds.
7. Serve and enjoy.

Nutrition:

Calories: 271 kcal

Fat: 3.7g

Carbs: 54g

Proteins: 6.5g

Coconut Pancakes

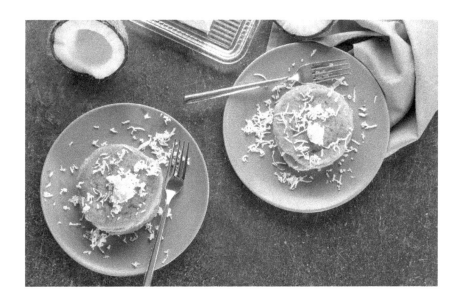

Preparation Time: 5 minutes

Cooking Time: 15 minutes

Servings: 4

Ingredients:

- ➤ 1 cup coconut flour
- ➤ 2 tbsps. arrowroot powder
- ➤ 1 tsp. baking powder
- ➤ 1 cup coconut milk
- ➤ 3 tbsps. coconut oil

Directions:

1. In a medium container, mix in all the dry ingredients.
2. Add the coconut milk and 2 tbsps. of the coconut oil then mix properly.
3. In a skillet, melt 1 tsp. of coconut oil.
4. Pour a ladle of the batter into the skillet then swirl the pan to spread the batter evenly into a smooth pancake.
5. Cook it for like 3 minutes on medium heat until it becomes firm.
6. Turn the pancake to the other side then cook it for another 2 minutes until it turns golden brown.
7. Cook the remaining pancakes in the same process.
8. Serve.

Nutrition:

Calories: 377 kcal

Fat: 14.9g

Carbs: 60.7g

Protein: 6.4g

Quinoa Porridge

Preparation Time: 5 minutes

Cooking Time: 25 minutes

Servings: 2

Ingredients:

- 2 cups coconut milk
- 1 cup rinsed quinoa
- 1/8 tsp. ground cinnamon
- 1 cup fresh blueberries

Directions:

1. In a saucepan, boil the coconut milk over high heat.
2. Add the quinoa to the milk then bring the mixture to a boil.
3. You then let it simmer for 15 minutes on medium heat until the milk is reduces.
4. Add the cinnamon then mix it properly in the saucepan.
5. Cover the saucepan and cook for at least 8 minutes until milk is completely absorbed.
6. Add in the blueberries then cook for 30 more seconds.
7. Serve.

Nutrition:

Calories: 271 kcal

Fat: 3.7g

Carbs: 54g

Protein:6.5g

Banana Barley Porridge

Preparation Time: 15 minutes

Cooking Time: 5 minutes

Servings: 2

Ingredients:

- 1 cup divided unsweetened coconut milk
- 1 small peeled and sliced banana
- 1/2 cup barley
- 3 drops liquid stevia
- 1/4 cup chopped coconuts

Directions:

1. In a bowl, properly mix barley with half of the coconut milk and stevia.
2. Cover the mixing bowl then refrigerate for about 6 hours.
3. In a saucepan, mix the barley mixture with coconut milk.
4. Cook for about 5 minutes on moderate heat.
5. Then top it with the chopped coconuts and the banana slices.
6. Serve.

Nutrition:

Calories: 159 kcal

Fat: 8.4g

Carbs: 19.8g

Proteins: 4.6g

Zucchini Muffins

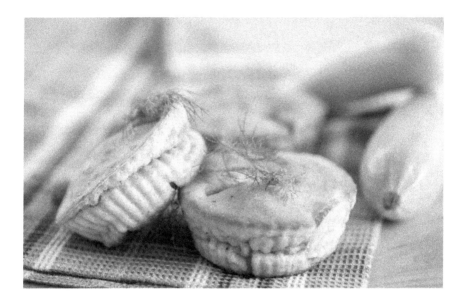

Preparation Time: 10 minutes

Cooking Time: 25 minutes

Servings: 16

Ingredients:

- 1 tbsp. ground flaxseed
- 3 tbsps. alkaline water
- 1/4 cup walnut butter
- 3 medium over-ripe bananas
- 2 small grated zucchinis
- 1/2 cup coconut milk
- 1 tsp. vanilla extract
- 2 cups coconut flour

- 1 tbsp. baking powder
- 1 tsp. cinnamon
- 1/4 tsp. sea salt

Directions:
1. Tune the temperature of your oven to 375°F.
2. Grease the muffin tray with the cooking spray.
3. In a bowl, mix the flaxseed with water.
4. In a glass bowl, mash the bananas then stir in the remaining ingredients.
5. Properly mix and then divide the mixture into the muffin tray.
6. Bake it for 25 minutes.
7. Serve.

Nutrition:

Calories: 127 kcal

Fat: 6.6g

Carbs: 13g

Protein: 0.7g

LUNCH

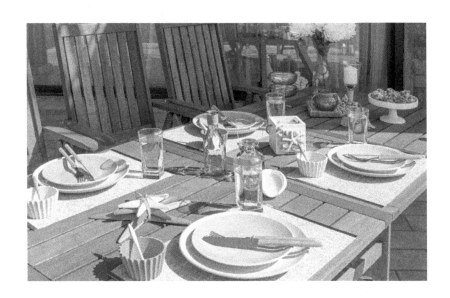

Chicken Loaf

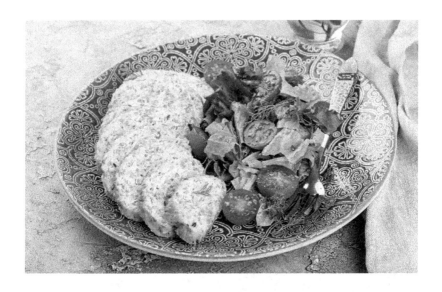

Preparation Time: 10 minutes

Cooking Time: 40 minutes

Servings: 4

Ingredients:

- 2 cups ground chicken
- 1 egg, beaten
- 1 tablespoon fresh dill, chopped
- 1 garlic clove, chopped
- ½ teaspoon salt
- 1 teaspoon chili flakes
- 1 onion, minced

Directions:

1. In the mixing bowl combine together all ingredient and mix up until you get smooth mass.
2. Then line the loaf dish with baking paper and put the ground chicken mixture inside.
3. Flatten the surface well.
4. Bake the chicken loaf for 40 minutes at 355°F.
5. Then chill the chicken loaf to the room temperature and remove from the loaf dish.
6. Slice it.

Nutrition:

Calories 167,

Fat 6.2 g,

Fiber 0.8 g,

Carbs 3.4 g,

Protein 32.2 g

Chicken Stroganoff

Preparation Time: 10 minutes

Cooking Time: 20 minutes

Servings: 4

Ingredients:

- 1 cup cremini mushrooms, sliced
- 1 onion, sliced
- 1 tablespoon olive oil
- ½ teaspoon thyme
- 1 teaspoon salt
- 1 cup Plain yogurt
- 10 oz chicken fillet, chopped

Directions:

1. Heat up olive oil in the saucepan.
2. Add mushrooms and onion.
3. Sprinkle the vegetables with thyme and salt. Mix up well and cook them for 5 minutes.
4. After this, add chopped chicken fillet and mix up well.
5. Cook the ingredients for 5 minutes more.
6. Then add plain yogurt, mix up well, and close the lid.
7. Cook chicken stroganoff for 10 minutes over the low heat.

Nutrition:

Calories 224,

Fat 9.2 g,

Fiber 0.8 g,

Carbs 7.4 g,

Protein 24.2 g

Lemon Caper Pesto

Preparation Time: 10 minutes

Cooking Time: 10 minutes

Servings: 1

Ingredients:

- 6 tablespoons fresh parsley leaves
- 3 cloves of garlic
- 2 tablespoons capers
- 2 oz. cashew nuts
- 2 tablespoons olive oil
- 1 tablespoon lemon juice

Directions:

1. Place all of the ingredients into a food processor and blitz until smooth.
2. Add a little extra oil if necessary.
3. Serve with pasta, vegetables, or meat dishes.

Nutrition:

Calories: 250

Sodium: 32 mg

Dietary Fibre: 1.6 g

Total Fat: 4.1 g

Total Carbs: 16.4 g

Protein: 1.5 g

Bacon Spaghetti Squash Carbonara

Preparation Time: 20 minutes

Cooking Time: 40 minutes

Servings: 4

Ingredients:

- 1 small spaghetti squash
- 6 ounces' bacon (roughly chopped)
- 1 large tomato (sliced)
- 2 chives (chopped)
- 1 garlic clove (minced)
- 6 ounces low-fat cottage cheese
- 1 cup Gouda cheese (grated)
- 2 tablespoons olive oil
- Salt and pepper, to taste

Directions:

1. Preheat the oven to 350°F.
2. Cut the squash spaghetti in half, brush with some olive oil and bake for 20–30 minutes, skin side up. Remove from the oven and remove the core with a fork, creating the spaghetti.
3. Heat one tablespoon of olive oil in a skillet. Cook the bacon for about 1 minute until crispy.
4. Quickly wipe out the pan with paper towels.

5. Heat another tablespoon of oil and sauté the garlic, tomato, and chives for 2–3 minutes. Add the spaghetti and sauté for another 5 minutes, occasionally stirring to keep from burning.
6. Begin to add the cottage cheese, about two tablespoons at a time. If the sauce becomes thick, add about a cup of water. The sauce should be creamy but not too runny or thick. Allow cooking for another 3 minutes.
7. Serve immediately.

Nutrition:

Calories: 305

Total Fat: 21 g

Net Carbs: 8 g

Protein: 18 g

Buttered Baked Cod with Wine

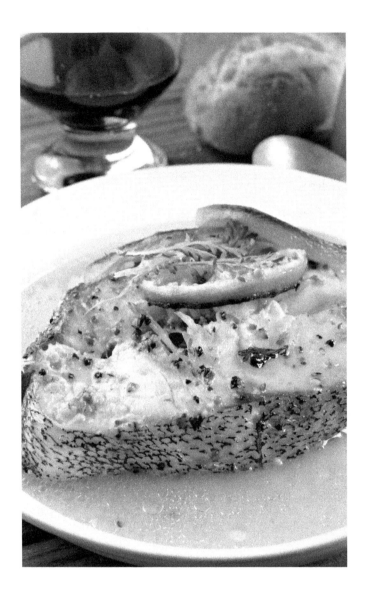

Preparation Time: 5 minutes

Cooking Time: 12 minutes

Servings: 2

Ingredients:

- 1 tablespoon butter
- 1 tablespoon butter
- 2 tablespoons dry white wine
- 1/2 pound thick-cut cod loin
- 1-1/2 teaspoons chopped fresh parsley
- 1-1/2 teaspoons chopped green onion
- 1/2 lemon, cut into wedges
- 1/4 sleeve buttery round crackers (such as Ritz®), crushed
- 1/4 lemon, juiced

Directions:

1. In a small bowl, melt butter in microwave. Whisk in crackers.
2. Lightly grease baking pan of air fryer with remaining butter. And melt for 2 minutes at 390°F.
3. In a small bowl whisk well lemon juice, white wine, parsley, and green onion.
4. Coat cod filets in melted butter. Pour dressing. Top with butter-cracker mixture.
5. Cook for 10 minutes at 390°F.
6. Serve and enjoy with a slice of lemon.

Nutrition:

Calories 266

Carbs: 9.3g

Protein: 20.9g

Fat: 16.1g

Spiced Sorghum and Berries

Preparation Time: 5 minutes

Cooking Time: 1 hour

Servings: 1

Ingredients:

- 1/4 cup whole-grain sorghum
- 1/4 teaspoon ground cinnamon
- 1/4 teaspoon Chinese five-spice powder
- 3/4 cups water
- 1/4 cup unsweetened nondairy milk
- 1/4 teaspoon vanilla extract
- 1/2 tablespoons pure maple syrup
- 1/2 tablespoon chia seed
- 1/8 cup sliced almonds
- 1/2 cups fresh raspberries, divided

Directions:

1. Using a large pot over medium-high heat, stir together the sorghum, cinnamon, five-spice powder, and water.
2. Wait for the water to a boil, cover it, and reduce the heat to medium-low.
3. Cook for one hour, or until the sorghum is soft and chewy. If the sorghum grains are still hard, add another cup of water and cook for 15 minutes more.

4. Using a glass measuring cup, whisk together the milk, vanilla, and maple syrup to blend.
5. Add the mixture to the sorghum and the chia seeds, almonds, and one cup of raspberries. Gently stir to combine.
6. When serving, top with the remaining one cup of fresh raspberries.

Nutrition:

Calories: 289

Fat: 8 g

Protein: 9 g

Carbohydrates: 52 g

Fiber: 10 g

Greek Salad

Preparation Time: 50 minutes

Cooking Time: 15 minutes

Servings: 5

Ingredients:

For Dressing:

- ½ teaspoon black pepper
- ¼ teaspoon salt
- ½ teaspoon oregano
- 1 tablespoon garlic powder
- 2 tablespoons Balsamic
- 1/3 cup olive oil

For Salad:

- ½ cup sliced black olives
- ½ cup chopped parsley, fresh
- 1 small red onion, thin-sliced
- 1 cup cherry tomatoes, sliced
- 1 bell pepper, yellow, chunked
- 1 cucumber, peeled, quarter and slice
- 4 cups chopped romaine lettuce
- ½ teaspoon salt
- 2 tablespoons olive oil

Directions:

1. In a small bowl, blend all of the ingredients for the dressing and let this set in the refrigerator while you make the salad.
2. To assemble the salad, mix together all the ingredients in a large-sized bowl and toss the veggies gently but thoroughly to mix.
3. Serve the salad with the dressing in amounts as desired

Nutrition:

Calories: 234,

Fat: 16.1 g,

Protein: 5 g,

Carbs: 48 g

Grilled Eggplants

Preparation Time: 10 minutes

Cooking Time: 10 minutes

Servings: 4

Ingredients:

- 1 large eggplant, cut into thick circles
- Salt and pepper to taste
- 1 tsp. smoked paprika
- 1 tbsp. coconut flour
- 1 tsp. lime juice
- 1 tbsp. olive oil

Directions:

1. Coat the eggplants in smoked paprika, salt, pepper, lime juice, coconut flour, and let it sit for 10 minutes.
2. In a grilling pan, add the olive oil.
3. Grill the eggplants for 3 minutes on each side.
4. Serve.

Nutrition:

Fat: 0.1 g

Sodium: 1.6 mg

Carbohydrates: 4.8 g

Fiber: 2.4 g

Sugars: 2.9 g

Protein: 0.8 g

Asparagus Avocado Soup

Preparation Time: 10 minutes

Cooking Time: 20 minutes

Servings: 4

Ingredients:

- 1 avocado, peeled, pitted, cubed
- 12 ounces asparagus
- ½ teaspoon ground black pepper
- 1 teaspoon garlic powder
- 1 teaspoon sea salt
- 2 tablespoons olive oil, divided
- 1/2 of a lemon, juiced
- 2 cups vegetable stock

Directions:

1. Switch on the air fryer, insert fryer basket, grease it with olive oil, then shut with its lid, set the fryer at 425 °F, and preheat for 5 minutes.
2. Meanwhile, place asparagus in a shallow dish, drizzle with 1tablespoon oil, sprinkle with garlic powder, salt, and black pepper, and toss until well mixed.
3. Open the fryer, add asparagus in it, close with its lid and cook for 10 minutes until nicely golden and roasted, shaking halfway through the frying.

4. When the air fryer beeps, open its lid and transfer asparagus to a food processor.
5. Add remaining ingredients into a food processor and pulse until well combined and smooth.
6. Tip the soup in a saucepan, pour in water if the soup is too thick, and heat it over medium-low heat for 5 minutes until thoroughly heated.
7. Ladle soup into bowls and serve.

Nutrition:

Calories: 208

Carbs: 2 g

Fat: 11 g

Protein: 4 g

Fiber: 5 g

Beer Battered Cod Filet

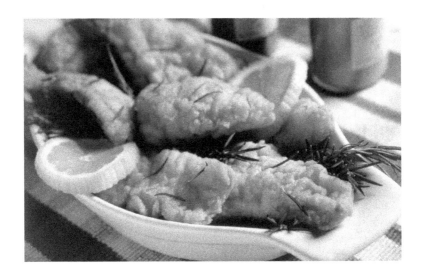

Preparation Time: 5 minutes

Cooking Time: 15 minutes

Servings: 2

Ingredients:

- ½ cup all-purpose flour
- ¾ teaspoon baking powder
- 1 ¼ cup lager beer
- 2 cod fillets
- 2 eggs, beaten
- Salt and pepper to taste

Directions:

1. Preheat the air fryer to 390°F.
2. Pat the fish fillets dry then set aside.
3. In a bowl, combine the rest of the Ingredients to create a batter.
4. Dip the fillets on the batter and place on the double layer rack.
5. Cook for 15 minutes.

Nutrition:

Calories 229

Carbs: 33.2g

Protein: 31.1g

Fat: 10.2g

Sweet Potato Chips

Preparation Time: 5 minutes

Cooking Time: 10 minutes

Servings: 4

Ingredients:

- 2 large sweet potatoes
- 15 ml. of oil
- 10 g of salt
- 2 g black pepper
- 2 g of paprika
- 2 g garlic powder
- 2 g onion powder

Directions:

1. Cut the sweet potatoes into strips 25 mm. thick.
2. Preheat the air fryer for a few minutes.
3. Add the cut sweet potatoes to a large bowl and mix with the oil until the potatoes are all evenly coated.
4. Sprinkle salt, black pepper, paprika, garlic powder, and onion powder. Mix well.
5. Place the French fries in the preheated baskets and cook for 10 minutes at 400 °F. Be sure to shake the baskets halfway through cooking.

Nutrition:

Calories: 123

Carbs: 2 g

Fat: 11 g

Protein: 4 g

Fiber: 0 g

Easy Beef Mushroom Stew

Preparation Time: 10 minutes

Cooking Time: 8 hours

Servings: 8

Ingredients:

- 2 lb stewing beef, cubed
- 1 packet dry onion soup mix
- 4 oz can mushrooms, sliced
- 14 oz can cream of mushroom soup
- 1/2 cup water
- 1/4 tsp black pepper
- 1/2 tsp salt

Directions:

1. Spray a crock pot inside with cooking spray.
2. Add all ingredients into the crock pot and stir well.
3. Cover and cook on low for 8 hours.
4. Stir well and serve.

Nutrition:

Calories 237

Fat: 5 g

Carbohydrates: 7 g

Sugar: 0.4 g

Protein: 31 g

Cholesterol: 101 mg

Béarnaise Sauce

Preparation Time: 5 minutes

Cooking Time: 3 minutes

Servings: 2

Ingredients:

- ½ cup butter
- 2 egg yolks, beaten
- 2 tsp. lemon juice, freshly squeezed
- ¼ tsp. onion powder
- 2 tbsp. fresh tarragon

Directions:

1. Press the SAUTÉ button on the Instant Pot.
2. Melt the butter for 3 minutes and transfer it into a mixing bowl.
3. While whisking the melted butter, slowly add the egg yolks.
4. Continue stirring so that no lumps form.
5. Add the lemon juice, onion powder, and fresh tarragon.
6. Serve.

Nutrition:

Calories: 603

Fat: 62 g

Carbs: 4 g

Protein: 5 g

Butterflied Prawns with Garlic-Sriracha

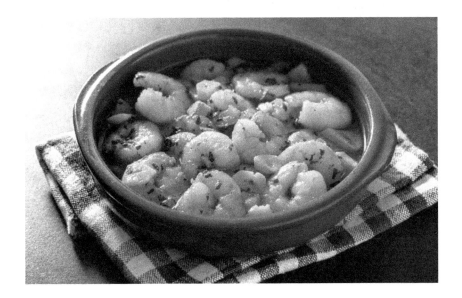

Preparation Time: 5 minutes

Cooking Time: 15 minutes

Servings: 2

Ingredients:

- 1 tablespoon lime juice
- 1 tablespoon sriracha
- 1-pound large prawns, shells removed and cut lengthwise or butterflied
- 1 teaspoon fish sauce
- 2 tablespoons melted butter
- 2 tablespoons minced garlic
- Salt and pepper to taste

Directions:

1. Preheat the air fryer to 390°F.
2. Place the grill pan accessory in the air fryer.
3. Season the prawns with the rest of the ingredients.
4. Place on the grill pan and cook for 15 minutes. Make sure to flip the prawns halfway through the cooking time.

Nutrition:

Calories : 443

Carbs: 9.7 g

Protein: 62.8g

Fat: 16.9g

Chili Sauce

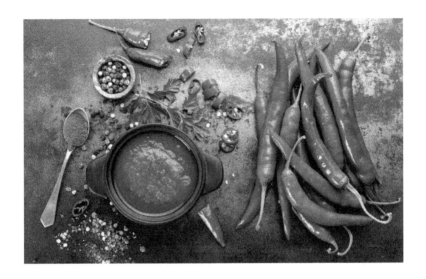

Preparation Time: 8 minutes

Cooking Time: 15 minutes

Servings: 2

Ingredients:

- 2 oz. hot peppers
- 2 cups of apple cider vinegar
- 1 tsp. salt

Directions:

1. Trim away the stems from the peppers and chop.
2. Add all ingredients to the Instant Pot.
3. Secure the lid and MANUALLY set the timer to 15 minutes under HIGH pressure.
4. Quick-release the pressure and serve the sauce into bowls.

Nutrition:

Calories: 2

Fat: 0 g

Carbs: 0.7 g

Protein: 1 g

Vanilla Caramel Sauce

Preparation Time: 5 minutes

Cooking Time: 13 minutes

Servings: 2

Ingredients:

- 2 tbsp. coconut oil
- 1 cup sugar
- 1 tsp vanilla extract
- 1/3 cup condensed coconut milk
- 1/3 cup water

Directions:

1. Warm up the Instant Pot using the SAUTÉ function.
2. Add the water and sugar, then stir and sauté for 13 minutes.
3. Stir in the milk, coconut oil, and vanilla.
4. Whisk until creamy and add to a glass container.
5. Cool completely and serve when ready.

Nutrition:

Calories: 80

Carbs: 14 g

Fat: 5 g

Protein: 0 g

Buffalo Chicken Soup

Preparation Time: 20 minutes

Cooking Time: 20 minutes

Servings: 4

Ingredients:

- 4 med. stalks celery, diced
- 2 med. carrots, diced
- 4 chicken breasts, boneless & skinless
- 6 tbsp. butter
- 1 qt. chicken broth
- 2 oz. cream cheese
- ½ c. heavy cream
- ½ c. buffalo sauce 1 tsp. sea salt
- ½ tsp. thyme, dried

For garnish:

- Sour cream
- Green onions, thinly sliced
- Bleu cheese crumbles

Direction:

1. Set a large pot to warm over medium heat with the olive oil in it.
2. Cook celery and carrot until shiny and tender. Add chicken breasts to the pot and cover. Allow cooking about five to six

minutes per side. Once the chicken has cooked and formed some caramelization on each side, remove it from the pot.

3. Shred the chicken breasts and set aside. Pour the chicken broth into the pot with the carrots and celery, then stir in the cream, butter, and cream cheese.
4. Bring the pot to a boil, then add chicken back to the pot. Stir buffalo sauce into the mix and combine completely. Feel free to increase or decrease as desired.
5. Add seasonings, stir, and drop the heat to low. Allow the soup to simmer for 15 to 20 minutes, or until all the flavors have fully combined. Serve hot with a garnish of sour cream, bleu cheese crumbles, and sliced green onion!

Nutrition:

Calories: 363

Carbohydrates: 4 grams

Fat: 32.5 grams

Protein: 57 grams

Cajun Seasoned Salmon Filet

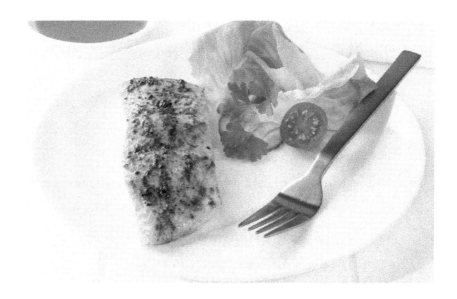

Preparation Time: 5 minutes

Cooking Time: 15 minutes

Servings: 1

Ingredients:

- 1 salmon fillet
- 1 teaspoon juice from lemon, freshly squeezed
- 3 tablespoons extra virgin olive oil
- A dash of Cajun seasoning mix
- Salt and pepper to taste

Directions:

1. Preheat the air fryer for 5 minutes.
2. Place all ingredients in a bowl and toss to coat.

3. Place the fish fillet in the air fryer basket.
4. Bake for 15 minutes at 3250F.
5. Once cooked drizzle with olive oil

Nutrition:

Calories 523

Carbohydrates: 4.6g

Protein: 47.9g

Fat: 34.8g

Chicken Fillets with Artichoke Hearts

Preparation Time: 10 minutes

Cooking Time: 30 minutes

Servings: 3

Ingredients:

- 1 can artichoke hearts, chopped
- 12 oz chicken fillets (3 oz each fillet)
- 1 teaspoon avocado oil
- ½ teaspoon ground thyme
- ½ teaspoon white pepper
- 1/3 cup water
- 1/3 cup shallot, roughly chopped
- 1 lemon, sliced

Directions:

1. Mix up together chicken fillets, artichoke hearts, avocado oil, ground thyme, white pepper, and shallot.
2. Line the baking tray with baking paper and place the chicken fillet mixture in it.
3. Then add sliced lemon and water.
4. Bake the meal for 30 minutes at 375F. Stir the ingredients during cooking to avoid burning.

Nutrition:

Calories 267,

Fat 8.2 g,

Fiber 3.8 g,

Carbs 10.4 g,

Protein 35.2 g

Chicken Meatballs with Carrot

Preparation Time: 10 minutes

Cooking Time: 10 minutes

Servings: 8

Ingredients:

- 1/3 cup carrot, grated
- 1 onion, diced
- 2 cups ground chicken
- 1 tablespoon semolina
- 1 egg, beaten
- ½ teaspoon salt
- 1 teaspoon dried oregano
- 1 teaspoon dried cilantro
- 1 teaspoon chili flakes
- 1 tablespoon coconut oil

Directions:

1. In the mixing bowl combine together grated carrot, diced onion, ground chicken, semolina, egg, salt, dried oregano, cilantro, and chili flakes.
2. With the help of scooper make the meatballs.
3. Heat up the coconut oil in the skillet.
4. When it starts to shimmer, put meatballs in it.
5. Cook the meatballs for 5 minutes from each side over the medium-low heat.

Nutrition:

Calories 107,

Fat 4.2 g,

Fiber 0.8 g,

Carbs 2.4 g,

Protein 11.2 g

Buttered Garlic-Oregano on Clams

Preparation Time: 5 minutes

Cooking Time: 5 minutes

Servings: 4

Ingredients:

- ¼ cup parmesan cheese, grated
- ¼ cup parsley, chopped
- 1 cup breadcrumbs
- 1 teaspoon dried oregano
- 2 dozen clams, shucked
- 3 cloves of garlic, minced
- 4 tablespoons butter, melted

Directions:

1. In a medium bowl, mix together the breadcrumbs, parmesan cheese, parsley, oregano, and garlic. Stir in the melted butter.
2. Preheat the air fryer to 390°F.
3. Place the baking dish accessory in the air fryer and place the clams.
4. Sprinkle the crumb mixture over the clams.
5. Cook for 5 minutes.

Nutrition:

    Calories: 160

    Carbs: 6.3g

    Protein: 2.9g

    Fat: 13.6g

DINNER

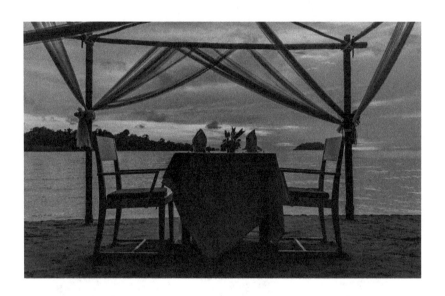

Thyme Scallops

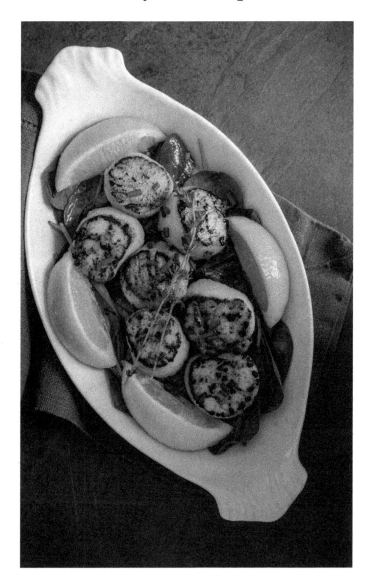

Preparation Time: 5 minutes

Cooking Time: 12 minutes

Servings: 1

Ingredients:

- 1 lb. scallops
- Salt and pepper
- ½ tbsp. butter
- ½ cup thyme, chopped

Directions:

1. Wash the scallops and dry them completely. Season with pepper and salt, then set aside while you prepare the pan.
2. Grease a foil pan in several spots with the butter and cover the bottom with the thyme. Place the scallops on top.
3. Pre-heat the fryer at 400°F and set the rack inside.
4. Place the foil pan on the rack and allow to cook for seven minutes.
5. Take care when removing the pan from the fryer and transfer the scallops to a serving dish. Spoon any remaining butter in the pan over the fish and enjoy.

Nutrition:

Calories: 291

Fat: 9g

Protein: 17g

Sugar: 5g

Oregano Pork Mix

Preparation Time: 5 minutes

Cooking Time: 7 hours and 6 minutes

Servings: 4

Ingredients:

- 2 pounds' pork roast
- 7 ounces' tomato paste
- 1 yellow onion, chopped
- 1 cup beef stock
- 2 tablespoons ground cumin
- 2 tablespoons olive oil
- 2 tablespoons fresh oregano, chopped
- 1 tablespoon garlic, minced
- ½ cup fresh thyme, chopped

Directions:

1. Heat up a sauté pan with the oil over medium-high heat, add the roast, brown it for 3 minutes on each side and then transfer to your slow cooker.
2. Add the rest of the ingredients, toss a bit, cover and cook on low for 7 hours.
3. Slice the roast, divide it between plates and serve.

Nutrition:

Calories: 623,

Fat 30.1 g

Fiber: 6.2 g

Carbs 19.3 g

Protein 69,2 g

Simple Beef Roast

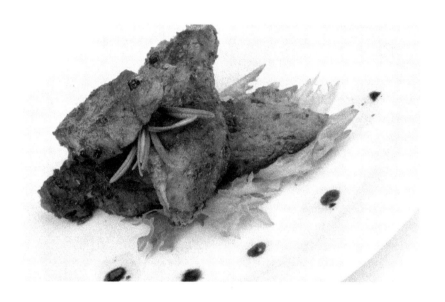

Preparation Time: 10 minutes

Cooking Time: 8 hours

Servings: 8

Ingredients:

- ➢ 5 pounds' beef roast
- ➢ 2 tablespoons Italian seasoning
- ➢ 1 cup beef stock
- ➢ 1 tablespoon sweet paprika
- ➢ 3 tablespoons olive oil

Directions:

1. In your slow cooker, mix all the ingredients, cover and cook on low for 8 hours.
2. Carve the roast, divide it between plates and serve.

Nutrition:

Calories: 587

Fat: 24.1 g

Fiber: 0.3 g

Carbs: 0.9 g

Protein: 86.5 g

Chicken Breast Soup

Preparation Time: 5 minutes

Cooking Time: 4 hours

Servings: 4

Ingredients:

- 3 chicken breasts, skinless, boneless, cubed
- 2 celery stalks, chopped
- 2 carrots, chopped
- 2 tablespoons olive oil
- 1 red onion, chopped
- 3 garlic cloves, minced
- 4 cups chicken stock
- 1 tablespoon parsley, chopped

Directions:

1. In your slow cooker, mix all the ingredients except the parsley, cover and cook on High for 4 hours.
2. Add the parsley, stir, ladle the soup into bowls and serve.

Nutrition:

Calories: 445

Fat: 21.1 g

Fiber: 1.6 g

Carbs: 7.4 g

Protein: 54,3 g

Cauliflower Curry

Preparation Time: 5 minutes

Cooking Time: 5 hours

Servings: 4

Ingredients:

- 1 cauliflower head, florets separated
- 2 carrots, sliced
- 1 red onion, chopped
- ¾ cup coconut milk
- 2 garlic cloves, minced
- 2 tablespoons curry powder
- A pinch of salt and black pepper
- 1 tablespoon red pepper flakes
- 1 teaspoon garam masala

Directions:

1. In your slow cooker, mix all the ingredients.
2. Cover, cook on high for 5 hours, divide into bowls and serve.

Nutrition:

Calories: 160

Fat: 11.5 g

Fiber: 5.4 g

Carbs: 14.7 g

Protein: 3,6 g

Tender & Juicy Lamb Roast

Preparation Time: 10 minutes

Cooking Time: 8 hours

Servings: 8

Ingredients:

- 4 lbs lamb roast, boneless
- ½ teaspoon thyme
- 1 teaspoon oregano
- 4 garlic cloves, cut into slivers
- ½ teaspoon marjoram
- ¼ teaspoon pepper
- 2 teaspoon salt

Directions:

1. Using a sharp knife make small cuts all over meat then insert garlic slivers into the cuts.
2. In a small bowl, mix together marjoram, thyme, oregano, pepper, and salt and rub all over lamb roast.
3. Place lamb roast into the slow cooker.
4. Cover and cook on low for 8 hours.
5. Serve and enjoy.

Nutrition:

Calories: 605

Fat: 48 g

Carbohydrates: 0.7 g

Sugar: 1 g

Protein: 36 g

Cholesterol: 160 mg

Basil Cheese Pork Roast

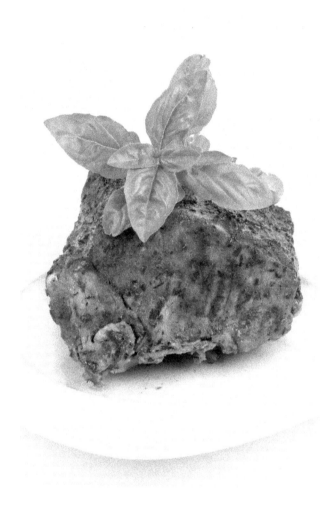

Preparation Time: 10 minutes

Cooking Time: 6 hours

Servings: 8

Ingredients:

- 2 lbs lean pork roast, boneless
- 1 teaspoon garlic powder
- 1 tablespoon parsley
- ½ cup cheddar cheese, grated
- 30 oz can tomatoes, diced
- 1 teaspoon dried oregano
- 1 teaspoon dried basil
- Pepper
- Salt

Directions:

1. Add the meat into the crock pot.
2. Mix together tomatoes, oregano, basil, garlic powder, parsley, cheese, pepper, and salt and pour over meat.
3. Cover and cook on low for 6 hours.
4. Serve and enjoy.

Nutrition:

Calories 260

Fat 9 g

Carbohydrates 5.5 g

Sugar 3.5 g

Protein 35 g

Cholesterol 97 mg

Feta Lamb Patties

Preparation Time: 10 minutes

Cooking Time: 12 minutes

Servings: 4

Ingredients:

- 1 lb ground lamb
- 1/2 teaspoon garlic powder
- 1/2 cup feta cheese, crumbled
- 1/4 cup mint leaves, chopped
- 1/4 cup roasted red pepper, chopped
- 1/4 cup onion, chopped
- Pepper
- Salt

Directions:

1. Add all ingredients into the bowl and mix until well combined.
2. Spray pan with cooking spray and heat over medium-high heat.
3. Make small patties from meat mixture and place on hot pan and cook for 6-7 minutes on each side.
4. Serve and enjoy.

Nutrition:

Calories 270

Fat 12 g

Carbohydrates 2.9 g

Sugar 1.7 g

Protein 34.9 g

Cholesterol 119 mg

Beef Stroganoff

Preparation Time: 10 Minutes

Cooking Time: 14 Minutes

Servings: 4

Ingredients:

- 9 Oz. Tender Beef
- 1 Onion, chopped
- 1 Tbsp. Paprika
- 3/4 Cup Sour Cream
- Salt and Pepper to taste
- Baking Dish

Directions:

1. Preheat the Cuisinart Air Fryer Oven to 390 degrees.
2. Chop the beef and marinate it using paprika.
3. Add the chopped onions into the baking dish and heat for about 2 minutes in the Cuisinart Air Fryer Oven.
4. Add the beef into the dish when the onions are transparent, and cook for 5 minutes.
5. Once the beef is starting to tender, pour in the sour cream and cook for another 7 minutes.
6. At this point, the liquid should have reduced. Season with salt and pepper and serve.

Nutrition:

    Calories: 254

    Fat: 21g

    Protein: 33g

    Fiber: 0g

Eggplant and Carrots Mix

Preparation Time: 5 minutes

Cooking Time: 25 minutes

Servings: 4

Ingredients:

- 1 pound eggplants, roughly cubed
- 1 pound baby carrots
- 1 cup heavy cream
- ½ teaspoon chili powder
- 1 teaspoon garlic powder
- 1 tablespoon chives, chopped
- A pinch of salt and black pepper

Directions:

1. In a pan that fits your air fryer, mix the eggplants with the carrots, cream and the other ingredients, toss, introduce in the air fryer and cook at 370 degrees F for 25 minutes.
2. Divide between plates and serve as a side dish.

Nutrition:

Calories: 129

Fat: 6 g

Fiber: 2 g

Carbs: 5 g

Protein 8 g

Parmesan Eggplants

Preparation Time: 5 minutes

Cooking Time: 20 minutes

Servings: 4

Ingredients:

- 1 pound eggplants, roughly cubed
- 1 tablespoon olive oil
- 1 teaspoon garlic powder
- 1 cup parmesan, grated
- A pinch of salt and black pepper
- Cooking spray

Directions

1. In the air fryer's pan, mix the eggplants with the oil and the other ingredients except the parmesan and toss.
2. Sprinkle the parmesan on top, put the pan in the machine and cook at 370 °F for 20 minutes.
3. Divide between plates and serve as a side dish.

Nutrition:

Calories: 183

Fat: 6 g

Fiber: 2 g

Carbs: 3 g

Protein: 8 g

Kale Sauté

Preparation Time: 5 minutes

Cooking Time: 15 minutes

Servings: 4

Ingredients:

- 1 tablespoon avocado oil
- 1 pound baby kale
- ½ cup heavy cream
- Salt and black pepper to the taste
- ¼ teaspoon chili powder
- 1 tablespoon dill, chopped
- ¼ cup walnuts, chopped

Directions

1. In a pan that fits the air fryer, mix the kale with the oil, cream and the other ingredients, toss, introduce the pan in the machine and cook at 360 °F for 15 minutes.
2. Divide between plates and serve as a side dish.

Nutrition:

Calories: 160

Fat: 7 g

Fiber: 2 g

Carbs: 4 g

Protein: 5 g

Carrots Sauté

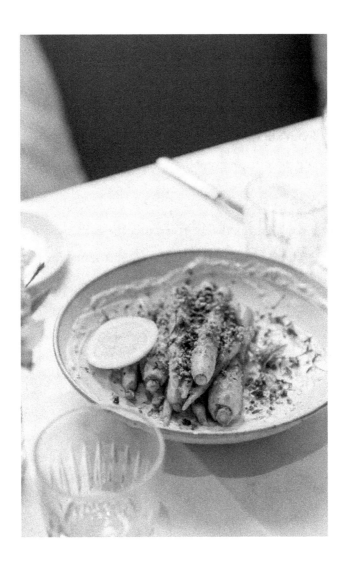

Preparation Time: 5 minutes

Cooking Time: 20 minutes

Servings: 4

Ingredients:

- 2 pounds baby carrots, peeled
- 1 tablespoon balsamic vinegar
- 2 tablespoons olive oil
- Salt and black pepper to the taste
- 1 tablespoon lemon juice
- 1/3 cup almonds, chopped
- ½ cup walnuts, chopped

Directions

1. In a pan that fits the air fryer, mix the carrots with the vinegar, oil and the other ingredients, toss, introduce the pan in the machine and cook at 380 °F for 20 minutes.
2. Divide between plates and serve as a side dish.

Nutrition:

Calories: 121

Fat: 9 g

Fiber: 2 g

Carbs: 4 g

Protein: 5 g

DESSERT

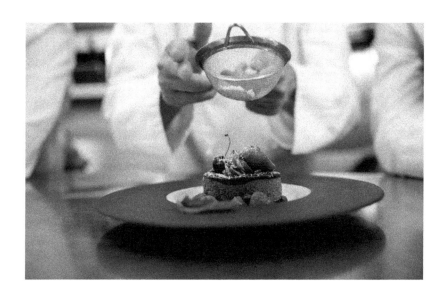

Almonds and Oats Pudding

Preparation Time: 10 minutes

Cooking Time: 15 minutes

Servings: 4

Ingredients:

- 1 tablespoon lemon juice
- Zest of 1 lime
- 1 and ½ cups almond milk
- 1 teaspoon almond extract
- ½ cup oats
- 2 tablespoons stevia
- ½ cup silver almonds, chopped

Directions:

1. In a pan, combine the almond milk with the lime zest and the other ingredients, whisk, bring to a simmer and cook over medium heat for 15 minutes.
2. Divide the mix into bowls and serve cold.

Nutrition:

Calories 174

Fat 12.1

Fiber 3.2

Carbs 3.9

Protein 4.8

Strawberry Sorbet

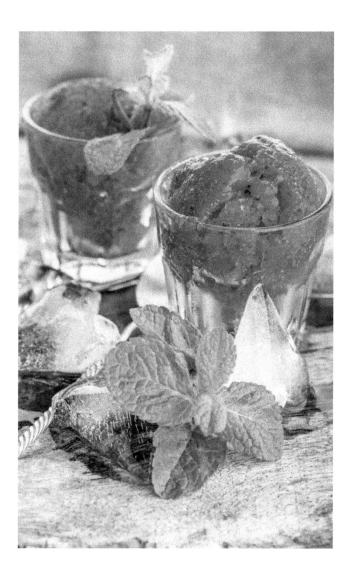

Preparation Time: 15 minutes

Cooking Time: 10 minutes

Servings: 6

Ingredients:

- 1 cup strawberries, chopped
- 1 tablespoon of liquid honey
- 2 tablespoons water
- 1 tablespoon lemon juice

Directions:

1. Preheat the water and liquid honey until you get homogenous liquid.
2. Blend the strawberries until smooth and combine them with honey liquid and lemon juice.
3. Transfer the strawberry mixture in the ice cream maker and churn it for 20 minutes or until the sorbet is thick.
4. Scoop the cooked sorbet in the ice cream cups.

Nutrition:

Calories 30,

Fat 0.4 g,

Fiber 1.4 g,

Carbs 14.9 g,

Protein 0.9 g

Chocolate Fondue

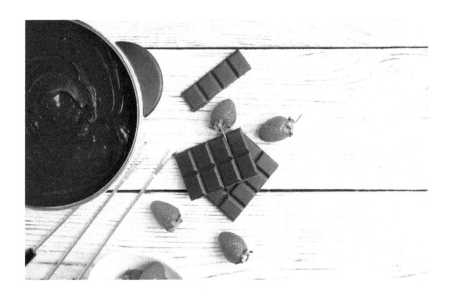

Preparation Time: 5 minutes

Cooking Time: 10 minutes

Servings: 2

Ingredients:

- 1 cup water
- ½ tsp. sugar
- ½ cup coconut cream
- ¾ cup dark chocolate, chopped

Directions:

1. Pour the water into your Instant Pot.
2. To a heatproof bowl, add the chocolate, sugar, and coconut cream.
3. Place in the Instant Pot.
4. Seal the lid, select MANUAL, and cook for 2 minutes. When ready, do a quick release and carefully open the lid. Stir well and serve immediately.

Nutrition:

Calories: 216

Fat: 17 g

Carbs: 11 g

Protein: 2 g

Rice Pudding

Preparation Time: 5 minutes

Cooking Time: 12 minutes

Servings: 2

Ingredients:

- ½ cup short grain rice
- ¼ cup of sugar
- 1 cinnamon stick
- 1½ cup milk
- 1 slice lemon peel
- Salt to taste

Directions:

1. Rinse the rice under cold water.
2. Put the milk, cinnamon stick, sugar, salt, and lemon peel inside the Instant Pot Pressure Cooker.
3. Close the lid, lock in place, and make sure to seal the valve. Press the PRESSURE button and cook for 10 minutes on HIGH.
4. When the timer beeps, choose the QUICK PRESSURE release. This will take about 2 minutes.
5. Remove the lid. Open the pressure cooker and discard the lemon peel and cinnamon stick. Spoon in a serving bowl and serve.

Nutrition:

Calories: 111

Fat: 6 g

Carbs: 21 g

Protein: 3 g

Braised Apples

Preparation Time: 5 minutes

Cooking Time: 12 minutes

Servings: 2

Ingredients:

- 2 cored apples
- ½ cup of water
- ½ cup red wine
- 3 tbsp. sugar
- ½ tsp. ground cinnamon

Directions:

1. In the bottom of Instant Pot, add the water and place apples.
2. Pour wine on top and sprinkle with sugar and cinnamon. Close the lid carefully and cook for 10 minutes at HIGH PRESSURE.
3. When done, do a quick pressure release.
4. Transfer the apples onto serving plates and top with cooking liquid.
5. Serve immediately.

Nutrition:

Calories: 245

Fat: 0.5 g

Carbs: 53 g

Protein: 1 g

Wine Figs

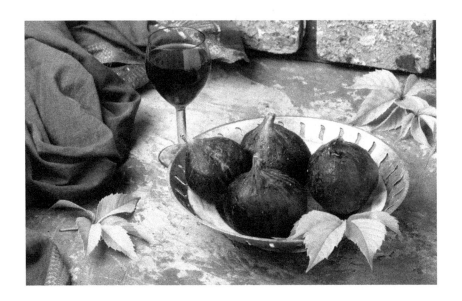

Preparation Time: 5 minutes

Cooking Time: 3 minutes

Servings: 2

Ingredients:

- ½ cup pine nuts
- 1 cup red wine
- 1 lb. figs
- Sugar, as needed

Directions:

1. Slowly pour the wine and sugar into the Instant Pot.
2. Arrange the trivet inside it; place the figs over it. Close the lid and lock. Ensure that you have sealed the valve to avoid leakage.
3. Press MANUAL mode and set timer to 3 minutes.
4. After the timer reads zero, press CANCEL and quick-release pressure.
5. Carefully remove the lid.
6. Divide figs into bowls, and drizzle wine from the pot over them.
7. Top with pine nuts and enjoy.

Nutrition:

Calories: 95

Fat: 3 g

Carbs: 5 g

Protein: 2 g

Olives and Cheese Stuffed Tomatoes

Preparation Time: 10 minutes

Cooking Time: 0 minutes

Servings: 24

Ingredients:

- 24 cherry tomatoes, top cut off and insides scooped out
- 2 tablespoons olive oil
- ¼ teaspoon red pepper flakes
- ½ cup feta cheese, crumbled
- 2 tablespoons black olive paste
- ¼ cup mint, torn

Directions:

1. In a bowl, mix the olives paste with the rest of the ingredients except the cherry tomatoes and whisk well.
2. Stuff the cherry tomatoes with this mix, arrange them all on a platter and serve as an appetizer.

Nutrition:

Calories 136;

Fat 8.6 g;

Fiber 4.8 g;

Carbs 5.6 g;

Protein 5.1 g

Tomato Salsa

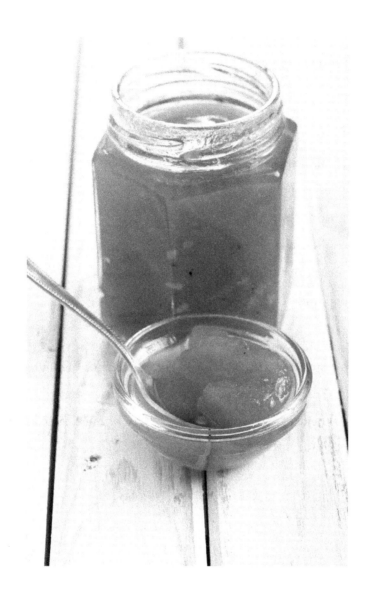

Preparation Time: 5 minutes

Cooking Time: 0 minutes

Servings: 6

Ingredients:

- 1 garlic clove, minced
- 4 tablespoons olive oil
- 5 tomatoes, cubed
- 1 tablespoon balsamic vinegar
- ¼ cup basil, chopped
- 1 tablespoon parsley, chopped
- 1 tablespoon chives, chopped
- Salt and black pepper to the taste
- Pita chips for serving

Directions:

1. In a bowl, mix the tomatoes with the garlic and the rest of the ingredients except the pita chips, stir, divide into small cups and serve with the pita chips on the side.

Nutrition:

Calories 160;

Fat 13.7 g;

Fiber 5.5 g;

Carbs 10.1 g;

Protein 2.2

Chili Mango and Watermelon Salsa

Preparation Time: 5 minutes

Cooking Time: 0 minutes

Servings: 12

Ingredients:

- 1 red tomato, chopped
- Salt and black pepper to the taste
- 1 cup watermelon, seedless, peeled and cubed
- 1 red onion, chopped
- 2 mangos, peeled and chopped
- 2 chili peppers, chopped
- ¼ cup cilantro, chopped
- 3 tablespoons lime juice
- Pita chips for serving

Directions:

2. In a bowl, mix the tomato with the watermelon, the onion and the rest of the ingredients except the pita chips and toss well.
3. Divide the mix into small cups and serve with pita chips on the side.

Nutrition:

Calories 62;

Fat 4g;

Fiber 1.3 g;

Carbs 3.9 g;

Protein 2.3 g

Apple Kale Cucumber Smoothie

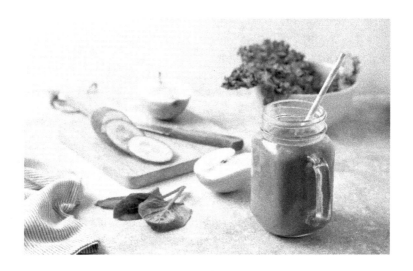

Preparation Time: 5 minutes

Cooking Time: 5 minutes

Servings: 1

Ingredients:

- ¾ cup water
- ½ green apple, diced
- ¾ cup kale
- ½ cucumber

Directions:

4. Toss all your ingredients into your blender then process till smooth and creamy.
5. Serve immediately and enjoy.

Nutrition:

Calories: 86
Fat: 0.5g
Carbs: 21.7g
Protein: 1.9g
Fiber: 0g

Cocoa Cake

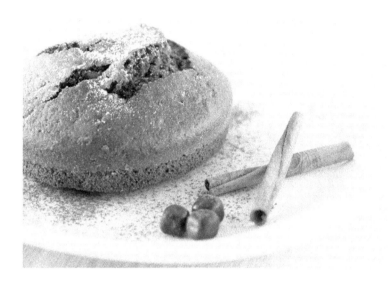

Preparation Time: 5 minutes

Cooking Time: 17 Minutes

Servings: 6

Ingredients:

- oz. butter
- 3 eggs
- 3 oz. sugar
- 1 tbsp. cocoa powder
- 3 oz. flour
- ½ tbsp. lemon juice

Directions:

1. Mix in 1 tablespoon butter with cocoa powder in a bowl and beat.
2. Mix in the rest of the butter with eggs, flour, sugar and lemon juice in another bowl, blend properly and move half into a cake pan
3. Put half of the cocoa blend, spread, add the rest of the butter layer and crest with remaining cocoa.
4. Put into air fryer and cook at 360° F for 17 minutes.
5. Allow to cool before slicing.
6. Serve.

Nutrition:

Calories: 221

Fat: 5g

Carbs: 12g

Apple Bread

Preparation Time: 5 minutes

Cooking Time: 40 Minutes

Servings: 6

Ingredients:

- 3 cups apples
- 1 cup sugar
- 1 tbsp. vanilla
- 2 eggs
- 1 tbsp. apple pie spice
- 2 cups white flour
- 1 tbsp. baking powder
- 1 stick butter
- 1 cup water

Directions:

1. Mix in egg with 1 butter stick, sugar, apple pie spice and turn using mixer.
2. Put apples and turn properly.
3. Mix baking powder with flour in another bowl and turn.
4. Blend the 2 mixtures, turn and move it to spring form pan.
5. Get spring form pan into air fryer and cook at 320°F for 40 minutes
6. Slice.
7. Serve.

Nutrition:

Calories: 401

Fat: 9g

Carbs: 29g

CONCLUSION

The Lean and Green diet's main aim is to help people reduce weight and obesity by controlled portion meals and snacks low in calories and carbohydrates.

Since the menu calls for eating carbs, protein, and healthy fat to be eaten, it is a reasonably healthy diet for healthy food. As far as weight reduction goes, experts agree that this program can benefit because its diet is low in calories, for the positive.

If you want to be successful with this diet you must:

- **Eat more fiber**: eat at least one serving of lean protein, healthy carbohydrates and a serving of fresh fruits and vegetables. Fiber does multiple things to the body, but for weight loss, it increases satiety to prevent over-eating, decreases the number of calories without feeling hungry all of the time, healthy fiber increases the metabolism of the body, cleans up the digestive system and you burn more calories.
- **Drink a lot of water**: the more water you drink, the more you get rid of the excess water. Drinking water will help you in eliminating unnecessary water from the body. To facilitate weight loss, drink at least 8 tall glasses of water a day.

And finally:

- **Do more exercise**: we must exercise as much as we know – just add some more minutes and increase the intensity. It's very important to move more and exercise on a regular basis if you want to keep your weight off.

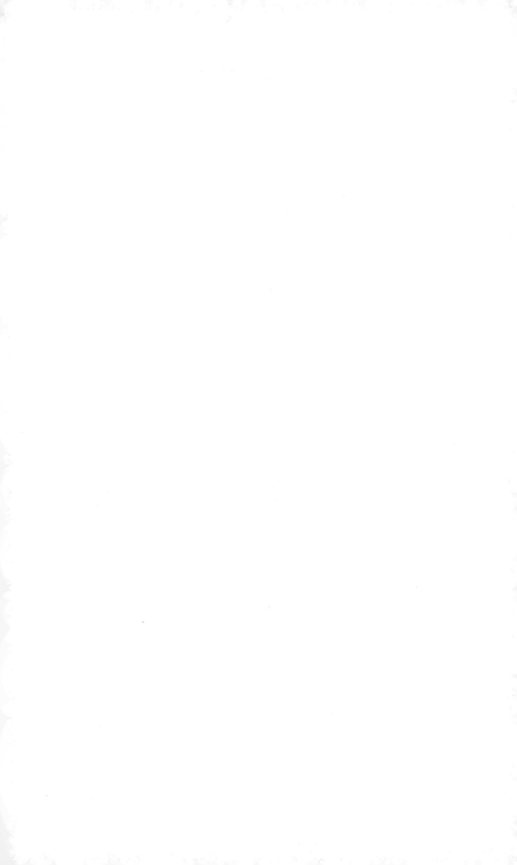

CPSIA information can be obtained
at www.ICGtesting.com
Printed in the USA
LVHW082106300321
682973LV00002B/62